Cancer-Fighting Recipes

Delicious and Nutritious Dishes to Help Lower Your Risk of Cancer

By

Linda A. ivey

Table of contents

Introduction

Cancer is a terrible illness that takes the lives of millions of people all over the globe. Diet is one of the most significant risk factors for developing cancer, despite the fact that there are many other variables that might play a role. According to a body of research, some foods and minerals have the potential to aid in the prevention of cancer and promote general health.

This cookbook's only purpose is to provide readers like you with delicious meals that are also high in nutrients and may help reduce the likelihood of developing cancer. We have made a great effort to select substances that are abundant in cancer-fighting elements, such as vitamins, minerals, antioxidants, and other micronutrients, and we have used them in our formulation. On the following pages, you will discover recipes for a variety of meals, including breakfast dishes, salads, soups, main dishes, sides, snacks, and desserts, all of which not only contribute to a healthy lifestyle but also have an excellent flavour. These dishes are guaranteed to please everyone at your dining party, whether you're preparing them for yourself, your family, or your friends.

Yet, eating is about more than simply the food that you place on your plate. It also depends on the manner in which food is prepared and the lifestyle that one leads. Because of this, we have included information on various changes in lifestyle that may assist in the prevention of cancer, in addition to guidelines for cooking and eating in a healthy manner.

I am of the opinion that everyone has the right to lead a life that is full of vitality and health, and it is my sincere wish that reading this book will assist you in working toward that objective. And with that, let's get started on the road to improved health and the prevention of cancer, one delicious meal at a time.

The Link Between Diet and Cancer

Cancer is a multifaceted illness that may be brought on by a wide variety of factors. Diet is a particularly crucial element in the development of cancer, according to a study. This is despite the fact that genetics, environmental factors, and lifestyle choices are all contributors to the disease.

According to the findings of many research, unhealthy eating habits and a lack of physical exercise are responsible for as much as one-third of all cancer fatalities that occur in the United States. This is due to the fact that some meals and nutrients have the ability to either encourage or discourage the formation of cancer cells. For instance, a diet that is heavy in processed and red meats has been connected to an increased risk of colorectal and other forms of cancer, while a diet that is high in fruits, vegetables, whole grains, and lean proteins has been associated with a decreased risk of cancer. [citation needed]

The relationship between one's food and their risk of developing cancer is intricate and multifaceted. Antioxidants and phytochemicals are two examples of the types of nutrients that have been shown to help protect cells from harm and prevent mutations that may lead to cancer. Certain others, including omega-3 fatty acids and fibre, have the potential to assist in the regulation of inflammation and the promotion of healthy cell development.

On the other hand, diets that are heavy in saturated and trans fats, sugar, and refined carbohydrates have been shown to induce inflammation, oxidative stress, and insulin resistance, all of which may contribute to the development of cancer.

It is essential to keep in mind that maintaining a healthy diet may help reduce the risk of developing cancer; nevertheless, this does not constitute a guarantee. There are a great number of additional variables that may play a role in the development of cancer, including genetics and environmental exposures.

Yet, if you want to reduce your risk of cancer and improve your general health and well-being, one of the most significant actions you can take is to make changes to your eating habits and adopt a healthier diet. You can help give your body the skills it needs to fight off cancer and other illnesses by including cancer-fighting foods and nutrients in your diet. This will help your body fight off cancer and other diseases.

Key Nutrients and Foods for Cancer Prevention
There are a number of essential nutrients and foods that have been shown to have qualities that are effective against cancer. The following are a few of the more significant ones:

- Antioxidants are molecules that help protect cells from damage produced by free radicals, which are known to contribute to the development of cancer. Antioxidants are known as antioxidants. Berries, citrus fruits, leafy greens, nuts, seeds, and other nuts and seeds are examples of foods that are rich in antioxidants.

- Fibre is essential for maintaining digestive health and supporting good bowel movements. Fibre is also crucial for sustaining digestive health. Fibre consumption has also been associated with a reduced likelihood of developing colorectal cancer. Whole grains, fruits, vegetables, and legumes are some examples of foods that are rich in fibre content.

- Omega-3 fatty acids: Omega-3 fatty acids are a form of good fat that has been related to a decreased risk of various different types of cancer, including breast, prostate, and colorectal cancers. This relationship has been shown via extensive research. Fatty fish (such as salmon and tuna), flaxseeds, and walnuts are examples of foods that are rich in omega-3 fatty acids. Other examples include walnuts.

- Cruciferous vegetables include substances that have been demonstrated to have anti-cancer qualities. Cruciferous vegetables include broccoli, cauliflower, kale, and cabbage, among others. These veggies have a high concentration of fibre in addition to other vital elements.

- Garlic: Compounds found in garlic have been demonstrated to have anti-cancer qualities, notably for stomach and colorectal malignancies. Garlic has been proven to have anti-cancer capabilities. In addition, studies have shown that eating garlic may reduce the chance of developing breast, lung, and prostate cancers.

- Catechins are found in green tea, which has been demonstrated to have anti-cancer qualities. Green tea also includes antioxidants called polyphenols. Many forms of cancer, including breast, prostate, and colorectal cancers, may have a lower incidence in those who consume green tea regularly, as this has been shown to be the case by several studies.

- Tomatoes: Tomatoes contain a chemical called lycopene, which has been related to a decreased risk of prostate cancer. In addition to this, tomatoes have a high concentration of vitamin C as well as other vital elements.

You may reduce your risk of cancer and improve your overall health and well-being by including certain foods and nutrients in your diet. This will help decrease your risk of cancer. Although you should do your best to consume a wide range of fruits, vegetables, whole grains, lean proteins, and healthy fats, you should try to cut down on processed and red meats, drinks with added sugar, and refined carbs. In addition, you may want to think about including some supplements in your diet in order to assist guarantee that you are receiving all of the necessary nutrients.

Tips for Eating and Cooking

The following are some dietary and culinary recommendations that may help lower your chance of developing cancer:

- Select foods that have been a little processed and are whole. Whole foods, such as fruits, vegetables, whole grains, and lean meats, are abundant in vital nutrients and are devoid of chemicals and preservatives that may be detrimental to one's health.

- Cook at home: When you cook at home, you have complete control over the materials and techniques of preparation that go into your meals. Experiment with different cancer-fighting products and nutritious meals to see what works best for you.

- Reduce your consumption of red and processed meats. Research has shown that eating red, and processed meats might raise your chance of developing some forms of cancer, including colorectal cancer. You should make an effort to cut down on your consumption of these meats and turn instead to sources of lean protein like chicken, fish, and plant-based foods.

- Consume a wide range of colourful fruits and vegetables. Fruits and vegetables of varying colours contain a variety of nutrients, some of which may reduce the risk of developing cancer. Eat foods that are different hues, such as blueberries, carrots, and spinach. This will help your body absorb more nutrients.

- Make use of healthy fats: Consuming healthy fats, such as those found in olive oil, avocados, and nuts, may assist in lowering inflammation and lowering the risk of developing cancer. You should make an effort to cut down on your consumption of bad fats like those found in fried meals and processed snacks.

- Reduce your use of alcohol since research has shown that drinking alcohol is associated with an increased risk of various forms of cancer, including breast and colorectal cancers. You should strive to consume no more than one alcoholic beverage per day if you are a woman and no more than two if you are a man.

- Sugary beverages, such as soda and sports drinks, have been associated with an elevated risk of numerous forms of cancer. To reduce this risk, you should avoid drinking sugary drinks. Instead, you should drink water or liquids that aren't sweetened.

- Increase your consumption of fibre: Consuming a diet rich in fibre has been associated with a decreased risk of numerous forms of cancer, including colorectal cancer. If you want to reduce your chance of developing cancer, this is an important factor to consider. In order to boost the amount of fibre you consume in your diet, it is important to consume a diet that is rich in fruits, vegetables, legumes, and whole grains.

- Green tea includes antioxidants and other substances that have been demonstrated to have cancer fighting qualities; thus, it is recommended that you drink green tea. If you want to reduce your risk of developing cancer, try drinking one or two cups of green tea every day.

- Certain spices, including turmeric and ginger, include anti-inflammatory properties that may help protect against cancer. Including these spices in your diet may help you avoid developing cancer. If you want to give your health a little more kick, try adding any of these spices to your meals or sipping some turmeric tea.

- When it is available, go for organic: There is evidence that pesticides and other chemicals used in standard agricultural techniques may raise a person's likelihood of developing cancer. If you want to cut down on your contact with harmful toxins, try to buy organic fruits and veggies whenever you can.

- Make use of ways that are healthful for cooking: The manner in which you prepare your food might also have an effect on the cancer-fighting capabilities it has, instead of frying or charbroiling your food, which may generate substances that are hazardous to your health, use healthier cooking techniques such as grilling, baking, or steaming instead.

- Controlling your portion sizes is important since eating too much of any meal, including nutritious foods, may cause you to gain weight and can raise your risk of developing many forms of cancer. Learn to limit your portions by measuring out your meals and paying attention to the indications your body gives you when it's hungry.

You may make modest adjustments to your lifestyle that, together, can have a significant positive effect on your health and lower your chance of developing cancer if you follow the advice shown here. Note that you should also discuss your unique risk factors with your physician, as well as any other preventative measures you may take against cancer.

Chapter 1

Breakfast and Brunch

Blueberry and Almond Butter Smoothie

A smoothie made with blueberries and almond butter is not only tasty but also a very healthy way to start the day. This smoothie will keep you feeling full and energetic all morning since it is loaded with cancer-fighting antioxidants, healthy fats, and protein. The following is the recipe for it:

Ingredients:

1 cup of blueberries from the freezer

One banana

One spoonful of butter made from almonds

1/2 cup almond milk

half a cup of Greek yoghurt

1 level teaspoon of honey (optional)

Instructions:

1. Put all of the ingredients into a blender and start blending.

2. Mix on high speed until the mixture is silky smooth and creamy.

3. Test it out, and if it's not sweet enough, sweeten it up with some honey.

4. Pour into a glass, and then sit back and enjoy!

5. This smoothie is not only tasty but also very nutritious since it contains a lot of different kinds of fruit. Anthocyanins are a kind of antioxidant that has been found to help protect against cancer, and blueberries are an excellent source of these anthocyanins. The almond butter that you buy at the store is a good source of protein, healthy fats, and vitamin E that has antioxidant characteristics. Greek yoghurt is an excellent source of protein and probiotics, both of which may help boost the immune system and promote digestive health.

Since it can be whipped together quickly and simply in a matter of minutes, this smoothie is an excellent choice for breakfast for those who are always on the go. It is also possible to tailor it to your preferences by using other nutrients that fight cancer, such as spinach or kale. Try out this dish for a nutritious and flavorful way to start your day, and you won't regret it!

This recipe does not specify the number of minutes since it may be mixed until it reaches the appropriate consistency. But, in most cases, blending for one to two minutes should be adequate to accomplish the desired silky and creamy consistency. If the smoothie is too thick, you may thin it out by adding a little more almond milk. On the other hand, if the smoothie is too thin, you can thicken it up by adding additional frozen blueberries or bananas. You should adjust the amount of time spent blending depending on your individual choice for the consistency and thickness of your smoothie.

Avocado Toast with Poached Eggs

Toast topped with avocado and eggs cooked in butter is a time-honoured morning meal that is not only tasty but also rich in nutrients that prevent cancer. The following is the recipe for it:

Ingredients:
Two pieces of bread made with all whole grains
One ripe avocado
Two big eggs

1/2 teaspoon of apple cider vinegar

To taste, salt and pepper are available.

Tomato slices, dried red pepper flakes, or fresh herbs may be used as a topping if desired.

Instructions:

1. Toast the bread pieces until they reach the amount of crispiness that you choose.
2. To prepare the avocado while the bread is toasting, split it in half lengthwise and remove the pit. The meat should be removed and placed in a basin before being mashed with a fork. Salt and pepper may be added to taste as a seasoning.
3. Put some water in a pot of around medium size, turn the heat up to medium, and bring the water to a low boil. Combine the water and vinegar in a bowl.
4. Separate one egg and place it in a ramekin or a small dish. Place the egg carefully into the water that is simmering, taking care to maintain the integrity of the white. Proceed in the same manner with the second egg.

5. The eggs should be poached for three to four minutes or until the whites have solidified, but the yolks have not.

6. Take the eggs out of the poaching liquid using a slotted spoon, and place them on a paper towel to dry off.

7. On the toasted bread pieces, spread the mashed avocado that you previously prepared.

8. Top each piece of bread with a poached egg and any extra toppings.

Serve right away, and have fun with it!

The preparation time for this dish ranges between ten and fifteen minutes, and it all depends on how browned you want the bread to become and how long it takes to poach the eggs. Yet, the time and effort are well worth it since not only is this meal tasty, but it is also an excellent dose of fibre, protein, and healthy fats. Although the poached eggs are a fantastic source of protein as well as other necessary elements, the avocado is loaded with monounsaturated fats and fibre. Eat this meal for breakfast or brunch and feed your day with cancer-fighting nourishment!

Greek Yogurt Parfait with Berries and Granola

Greek yoghurt parfait with berries and granola is a healthy and delicious breakfast or snack that's packed with cancer-fighting nutrients. Here's how to make it:

Ingredients:

1 cup plain Greek yoghurt

1/2 cup mixed berries (such as strawberries, blueberries, and raspberries)

1/4 cup granola

One tablespoon honey (optional)

Instructions:

1. Rinse the berries and slice any larger ones into bite-sized pieces.
2. In a glass or bowl, layer the Greek yoghurt, mixed berries, and granola.
3. Repeat the layers until all the ingredients are used up, ending with a layer of granola on top.
4. Drizzle with honey, if desired.
5. Serve immediately and enjoy!
6. This recipe takes approximately 5-10 minutes to prepare, depending on how much time you spend

slicing the berries and layering the ingredients. It's a great breakfast or snack option that's not only easy to make but also packed with cancer-fighting nutrients. Greek yoghurt is a great source of protein and probiotics, while berries are a rich source of antioxidants and fibre. Granola adds a satisfying crunch and is a good source of fibre, healthy fats, and protein. Customize this recipe by using your favourite type of berry or granola, and enjoy a nutritious and delicious meal or snack anytime!

Spinach and Mushroom Frittata

The frittata with spinach and mushrooms is a delicious dish that can be enjoyed for every meal of the day, including breakfast, lunch, and even supper. The following is the recipe for it:

Ingredients:
Six big eggs
1/4 cup milk
1/4 teaspoon salt 1/4 teaspoon black pepper
One tablespoon of olive oil
half a cup of mushroom slices

Two cups of spinach leaves that are still young.

1/4 cup of feta cheese in crumbled form (optional)

Instructions:

1. Turn the oven up to 350 degrees Fahrenheit.
2. Eggs, milk, salt, and black pepper should be mixed together in a large basin using a whisk.
3. Olive oil should be heated in a big pan that may go in the oven over medium heat.
4. Sauté the sliced mushrooms for around three to four minutes or until they begin to lose their firmness.
5. Put the young spinach leaves in the pan and cook them over medium heat, tossing them regularly until they become wilted.
6. After pouring the egg mixture into the pan, give it a little toss to ensure that the veggies are uniformly distributed.
7. If used, crumbled feta cheese should be sprinkled over the top at this point.
8. When the oven has been prepared, place the pan inside and bake the frittata for around 15 to 20 minutes, or until it is firm in the middle and golden brown around the edges.

9. Take the pan out of the oven and wait a few minutes
    for the frittata to cool completely before slicing it and
    serving it.

The preparation time for this dish ranges between thirty and forty minutes, depending on how long it takes to bake the frittata and sauté the veggies called for in the recipe. Including mushrooms and leafy greens in your diet is a fantastic method to increase your consumption of cancer-fighting elements like antioxidants, fibre, and vitamins, each of which is abundant in these foods. It is possible to make this dish vegan or dairy-free by omitting feta cheese, which, in addition to contributing a tangy taste, is an excellent source of calcium and protein. At any time of the day, this frittata filled with spinach and mushrooms will provide you with a meal that is both nourishing and gratifying.

Egg scramble

A scrambled egg breakfast is a meal that can be made in a short amount of time and is simple to personalize by adding the veggies, herbs, and spices of your choice. The following is the recipe for it:

Ingredients:

Three big eggs

1/4 cup milk

1/4 teaspoon salt 1/4 teaspoon black pepper

One tablespoon of butter or olive oil

0.5 grams of finely chopped veggies (such as bell peppers, onions, mushrooms, and spinach)

a quarter of a cup of shredded cheese (optional)

Instructions:

1. Eggs, milk, salt, and black pepper should be mixed together in a small bowl using a whisk until they are completely incorporated.

2. Warm the butter or olive oil in a skillet that does not cling to the pan by placing it over medium-high heat.

3. When the veggies have been chopped, add them to the pan and sauté them for about two to three minutes or until they begin to soften.

4. After pouring the egg mixture into the pan, give it a little toss to ensure that the veggies are uniformly distributed.

5. Cook the eggs for two to three minutes, swirling the pan regularly until the whites are set but the yolks are still runny.

6. If you are using shredded cheese, sprinkle it over the top of the dish, and then heat it for an additional one to two minutes or until the cheese is melted and bubbling.

7. Take the egg scramble off the heat, and serve it in the skillet while it's still hot.

The preparation time for this dish is anywhere from ten to fifteen minutes, depending on how quickly the veggies can be chopped and how quickly the eggs can be cooked. It is an excellent method for including veggies and protein into one's diet, both of which are essential for the avoidance of cancer. You may make this dish your own by substituting the veggies listed above with others of your choosing, such as tomatoes cut into cubes, sliced zucchini, or chopped kale. In addition to contributing additional taste and nutrition, fresh herbs such as parsley, basil, or cilantro may also be used. For a healthier and lighter version of this meal, omit the cheese altogether or use just a tiny quantity. Scrambled eggs are a great option for a quick and filling breakfast or brunch dish.

Chapter 2

Salads and Appetizers

Rainbow Salad with Grilled Chicken and Citrus Dressing

The Rainbow Salad with Grilled Chicken and Citrus Dressing is a vibrant salad that is high in nutrients and is excellent for either lunch or supper. This salad is packed with a wide range of cancer-fighting veggies, fruits, and lean protein sources, making it an excellent choice for a dinner that is both nutritious and satisfying.

Ingredients:

1 pound of chicken breasts that are boneless and skinless

6 cups of a variety of greens (such as kale, spinach, and arugula)

1 tbsp. of red cabbage that has been chopped

1 ounce of carrots, chopped

One standard measuring cup of chopped red bell pepper

One standard measuring cup of diced yellow bell pepper

1 ounce of diced mango

1/4 cup of fresh cilantro that has been chopped

a quarter of a cup of sliced almonds

To taste, salt and black pepper will be used.

For the Dressing Made with Citrus:

1/4 of a cup of freshly squeezed orange juice

1/4 cup fresh lemon juice

Two measuring teaspoons of honey

Two tablespoons extra-virgin olive oil

One teaspoon of Dijon mustard

To taste, salt and black pepper will be used.

Instructions:

1. Prepare the grill for cooking over medium-high heat. Add some salt and black pepper to the chicken breasts, and set them aside.

2. If you want the chicken breast to have an internal temperature of 165 degrees Fahrenheit, grill it for 6 to 8 minutes on each side. Before cutting it, give it a five-minute rest first.

3. Mix the mixed greens, red cabbage, carrots, red bell pepper, yellow bell pepper, mango, and cilantro together in a large bowl.

4. To prepare the dressing, put the orange juice, lemon juice, honey, olive oil, Dijon mustard, salt, and black pepper into a small bowl and mix all of the ingredients together.

5. After pouring the dressing over the salad, give it a little toss to distribute it evenly.

6. After dividing the salad among serving dishes, garnish each bowl with sliced almonds and chicken that has been grilled.

7. As soon as possible, serve the Rainbow Salad topped with Grilled Chicken and Citrus Dressing.

The preparation time for this dish is around half an hour, and it makes enough food for four servings. The vibrant veggies and fruits that make up this salad are an excellent source of a wide variety of vitamins, minerals, fibre, and antioxidants, and the grilled chicken that tops it is an excellent amount of protein. The citrus dressing contributes a taste that is both zesty and acidic, which is a nice contrast to the sweetness of the mango.

Greek Salad:

2 cups chopped romaine lettuce

1/2 cup of cucumber that has been chopped.

1/2 cup of tomato pieces, chopped

a quarter of a cup of chopped red onion and a quarter of a cup

of sliced kalamata olives

1/4 cup of feta cheese in crumbled form (optional)

Two tablespoons extra-virgin olive oil

One tablespoon of vinegar made from red wine

Oregano, dry, one-fourth of a teaspoon

To taste, salt and black pepper will be used.

Instructions:

1. Mix the chopped lettuce, cucumber, tomato, and red onion with the olives in a big bowl. Add in the olives.

2. To create the dressing, put the olive oil, red wine vinegar, dried oregano, salt, and black pepper into a small dish and whisk all of the ingredients together.

3. After pouring the dressing over the salad, give it a little toss to distribute it evenly.

4. If used, crumbled feta cheese should be sprinkled over the top at this point.

The Greek salad should be served cold.

The preparation time for this meal is around ten to fifteen minutes, depending on how quickly the veggies may be chopped. Because of the olives and the olive oil, it is an excellent source of fibre as well as antioxidants and healthy fats.

Hummus and Vegetable Platter:

1 ounce of hummus

1 cup of raw veggies of varying types (such as carrots, celery, bell peppers, and cherry tomatoes)

1/4 cup pitted kalamata olives

1/4 cup of feta cheese in crumbled form (optional)

Instructions:

1. Position the hummus so that it is in the middle of a big dish.
2. Arrange the raw veggies, olives, and feta cheese around the hummus if you'd like to use any of those ingredients.
3. The hummus and vegetable dish should be served cold.
4. The preparation time for this meal is around ten to fifteen minutes, depending on how quickly the

veggies may be chopped. It is an excellent method for obtaining a wide range of vitamins, minerals, and pigments from the veggies, in addition to the protein and fibre that may be obtained from the hummus.

Tomato, and then some Basil

Bruschetta is made using one loaf of French bread that has been sliced and two teaspoons of extra-virgin olive oil.

One clove of garlic, finely chopped
1 cup chopped tomato
1/4 cup of fresh basil that has been chopped
To taste, salt and black pepper will be used.

Instructions:

- Turn the oven up to 350 degrees Fahrenheit.
- Olive oil should be used to brush the sliced bread, which should then be placed on a baking pan.
- Toast the bread in the oven for five to seven minutes or until it is just slightly golden.
- To prepare the topping, mix the minced garlic, diced tomato, chopped basil, kosher salt, and freshly ground black pepper in a small bowl.

- Place a dollop of the tomato and basil mixture on each piece of toasted bread.
- You may serve the bruschetta with the tomato and basil warm or at room temperature.

The preparation time for this dish ranges anywhere from ten to fifteen minutes, depending on how quickly the veggies can be chopped and how quickly the bread can be toasted. In addition to the heart-healthy advantages of olive oil, this is an excellent method for appreciating the savoury tastes of fresh tomatoes and basil.

Quinoa Salad with Roasted Vegetables

1 ounce of ready-to-eat quinoa

1 cup of veggies that have been roasted (such as bell peppers, zucchini, eggplant, and onions)

1/4 cup of fresh parsley that has been chopped

1/4 cup of feta cheese in crumbled form (optional)

Two tablespoons extra-virgin olive oil

One tablespoon of lemon juice

1 milligram (mg) of honey

To taste, salt and black pepper will be used.

Instructions:

1. Mix together the quinoa that has been cooked, the roasted vegetables, the chopped parsley, and the crumbled feta cheese, if using, in a large bowl.

2. To create the dressing, put the olive oil, lemon juice, honey, salt, and black pepper into a small bowl and mix all of the ingredients together.

3. After pouring the dressing over the quinoa salad, give it a little toss to distribute it evenly.

4. The quinoa salad should be served cold.

5. Preparing this dish might take anywhere from thirty to forty minutes, depending on how long it takes the quinoa to cook and how long the veggies take to roast. Because of the quinoa and the veggies, this dish is an excellent source of protein, fibre, and vitamins.

Broccoli and Cauliflower Salad with Dried Cranberries and Walnuts

The Broccoli and Cauliflower Salad with Dried Cranberries and Walnuts is a nutritious and delectable salad that is ideal for a light lunch or as a side dish for supper since it is both of those things. This salad is chock full of cruciferous veggies, which have been shown to reduce the risk of cancer, as well as almonds and dried cranberries, which are high in antioxidants.

Ingredients:

4 cups of broccoli florets that have been chopped

4 cups of cauliflower florets that have been chopped

1/4 cup of finely sliced crimson onion

Cranberries, dried, one-half cup

1/2 cup of walnuts that have been chopped

1/4 cup apple cider vinegar

Two measuring teaspoons of honey

Two teaspoons of Dijon mustard

1/4 cup extra-virgin olive oil

To taste, salt and black pepper will be used.

Instructions:

1. Mix the broccoli florets, cauliflower florets, red onion, dried cranberries, and chopped walnuts together in a large basin.
2. To prepare the dressing, put the apple cider vinegar, honey, Dijon mustard, olive oil, salt, and black pepper

into a small bowl and mix all of the ingredients together.

3. After pouring the dressing over the salad, give it a little toss to distribute it evenly.

4. Before serving, place the salad in the refrigerator for at least half an hour to enable the flavours to come together.

5. It is best to refrigerate the Broccoli and Cauliflower Salad with Dried Cranberries and Walnuts before serving.

The preparation time for this dish is roughly twenty minutes, and it makes enough food for four servings. The cruciferous vegetable broccoli and cauliflower both contain sulforaphane, a chemical that research has shown to have anti-cancer characteristics. Sulforaphane is found in both of these plants. The walnuts and dried cranberries not only provide a satisfying crunch and a natural sweetness to the salad, but they are also an excellent source of antioxidants and healthy fats. The taste of veggies and fruits in the salad is complemented by the dressing, which is acidic and has a hint of sweetness.

Smoked salmon and cucumber bites

One peeled and sliced cucumber, 4 ounces of cured salmon

a quarter of a cup of whipped cream cheese

One tablespoon of fresh dill that has been chopped

To taste, salt and black pepper will be used.

Instructions:

- Put the cucumber slices on a dish that's meant for serving.
- After cutting up into bite-sized pieces, the smoked salmon should be placed on top of the cucumber slices.
- Combine the whipped cream cheese, the chopped dill, the salt, and the black pepper in a small bowl and stir well.
- On top of each salmon and cucumber bite, dollop a little dab of the cream cheese mixture that has been mixed together.
- Chill the cucumber bites and smoked salmon appetizers before serving.

The preparation time for this meal is roughly ten to fifteen minutes. Because of the smoked salmon and the cucumber, it is an excellent source of protein, as well as beneficial fats and vitamins.

In general, eating cancer-fighting meals like salads and appetizers may be a delicious and healthful approach to including such items in your diet. These dishes are simple to put together and may either stand alone as snacks or be included in larger meals.

Chapter 3

Soups and Stews

Dishes such as soups and stews are not only nourishing but also soothing, and they may simply be loaded with components that fight cancer. They are also adaptable and may be altered to suit your own tastes in terms of flavour. The following are some recipes for nutritious and delicious soups and stews that you may make at home.

Butternut Squash and Carrot Soup

Ingredients

One butternut squash, peeled and cut into cubes, medium size

Four big carrots, peeled and chopped into small pieces.

One medium-sized onion, finely chopped

4 cups of broth made from vegetables

Two tablespoons of olive oil

To taste, salt and black pepper will be used.

Additional toppings, if desired: croutons, chopped parsley, or pumpkin seeds with croutons also work.

Instructions:

1. The olive oil should be heated in a large saucepan over medium heat.
2. After adding the chopped onion, continue to sauté for another 5 minutes until the onion is tender.
3. Place the carrots and butternut squash cubes into the saucepan, and swirl to mix the ingredients.
4. After the vegetable broth has been added, the mixture should be brought to a boil.
5. Turn the heat down to a low setting and allow the soup to simmer for twenty minutes or until the veggies have reached the desired level of doneness.
6. You may purée the soup until it is smooth using an immersion blender or by transferring it to a blender.
7. Salt and black pepper should be added to taste before eating the soup.
8. If you choose, you may garnish the hot Butternut Squash and Carrot Soup with chopped parsley, pumpkin seeds, or croutons. The soup should be served hot.

The preparation time for this dish is roughly thirty-five minutes, and it makes enough food for four servings. Carrots and butternut squash both contain high levels of beta-carotene, a kind of carotenoid that has been linked to a lower risk of developing some forms of cancer.

Chicken and Vegetable Stew

Ingredients:

1 pound of boneless, skinless chicken breasts, cut into 1-inch cubes one big onion, chopped three garlic cloves, minced two large carrots, peeled and chopped two celery stalks, chopped one can of diced tomatoes one can of water one can of chicken broth

4 cups of chicken broth with a reduced sodium content

One teaspoon of thyme in its dry form

One teaspoon of oregano that has been dried

To taste, salt and black pepper will be used.

Additional toppings, if desired: grated Parmesan cheese or minced parsley may be added.

Instructions:

1. One tablespoon of olive oil should be heated in a big saucepan set over medium heat.

2. Sauté the chopped onion and minced garlic in the saucepan until the onion is tender and transparent. Add the chopped onion to the pot.

3. When the chicken has been browned on both sides, add the chicken cubes to the saucepan and continue to simmer.

4. Place the chopped carrots, celery, tomato chunks, diced tomatoes, thyme, and oregano into the saucepan. Stir to combine.

5. Bring the mixture to a boil, then immediately decrease the heat to a low setting and allow the stew to simmer for thirty to forty minutes, or until the veggies are soft and the chicken is cooked through.

6. Salt and black pepper should be added to taste before eating the stew.

7. Serve the Chicken and Vegetable Stew while it is still hot, and if you want, sprinkle it with some chopped parsley or grated Parmesan cheese.

The preparation time for this dish is around half an hour, and it makes enough food for four servings. Although veggies give fibre, vitamins, and minerals that are essential for general health and cancer prevention, chicken delivers lean protein.

Lentil Soup

Ingredients

1 cup of lentils, either green or brown, that has been dried, rinsed, and drained

One big chopped onion, three garlic cloves minced, two carrots peeled and chopped, two celery stalks chopped, 4 cups of vegetable broth with a reduced sodium content

One teaspoon of cumin that has been ground

One teaspoon of coriander that has been ground

To taste, salt and black pepper will be used.

Additional toppings, if desired: fresh parsley that has been chopped, a touch of olive oil, or a few drops of fresh lemon juice

Instructions:

1. One tablespoon of olive oil should be heated in a big saucepan set over medium heat.

2. Sauté the chopped onion and minced garlic in the saucepan until the onion is tender and transparent. Add the chopped onion to the pot.

3. Add the chopped carrots and celery to the saucepan, then heat for another three to four minutes or until the vegetables have become somewhat softer.

4. After rinsing the lentils, add them to the saucepan along with the vegetable broth, cumin, coriander, salt, and black pepper. Stir everything together.

5. Bring the mixture to a boil, then immediately decrease the heat to a low setting and allow the soup to simmer for thirty to forty minutes, or until the lentils are soft and the soup has thickened.

6. Salt and black pepper should be added to taste after adjusting the seasoning.

7. The Lentil Soup may be served hot, garnished with chopped fresh parsley, a drizzle of olive oil, or a squeeze of lemon juice, depending on your personal preference.

The preparation time for this dish is around half an hour, and it makes enough food for four servings. The plant-based protein, fibre, and a number of cancer-fighting elements, such as folate, iron, and polyphenols, that can be found in lentils make them an excellent food source.

Beef and Barley Stew

Ingredients

1 pound of beef stew meat, chopped into tiny cubes, to be used in the stew

One big chopped onion, three garlic cloves minced, two carrots peeled and sliced, two celery stalks cut, 1 cup chopped water chestnuts

1 cup pearl barley

4 cups of beef broth with a reduced sodium content

One teaspoon of thyme in its dry form

One bay leaf

To taste, salt and black pepper will be used.

Additional toppings, if desired: grated Parmesan cheese or chopped fresh parsley may be added.

Instructions:

1. One tablespoon of olive oil should be heated in a big saucepan set over medium heat.

2. After the meat has been browned on both sides, remove it from the saucepan and set it aside.

3. Sauté the chopped onion and minced garlic in the saucepan until the onion is tender and transparent. Add the chopped onion to the pot.

4. Place the diced carrots, celery, and pearl barley in the saucepan along with the thyme, bay leaf, and beef broth. Stir to mix all of the ingredients.

5. Bring the mixture to a boil, then immediately turn the heat down to low and let the stew simmer for an additional one to one and a half hours, or until the beef is fork-tender and the barley is fully cooked.

6. After removing the bay leaf from the saucepan, season the stew to taste with salt and freshly ground black pepper.

7. If you want, you may top the beef and barley stew with some freshly chopped parsley or some grated Parmesan cheese before serving it hot.

The preparation time for this meal is roughly two to two and a half hours, and it serves four people. Barley is a wonderful source of fibre as well as various vitamins and minerals that are crucial for the prevention of cancer, and beef is an excellent source of protein and iron.

Vegetable and Lentil Soup with Kale and Tomatoes

Ingredients:

1 cup of brown lentils, which have been dried, rinsed, and drained

One chopped onion three minced garlic cloves two chopped carrots two chopped celery stalks 2 cups of low-sodium vegetable broth one chopped onion three minced garlic cloves one chopped carrot two chopped celery stalks one chopped onion 1 cup

One can of diced tomatoes, which have not been drained.

2 cups of kale leaves that have been chopped

One teaspoon of thyme in its dry form

One teaspoon of smoked paprika

To taste, salt and black pepper will be used.

Additional toppings, if desired: fresh parsley that has been chopped, a touch of olive oil, or a few drops of fresh lemon juice

Instructions:

1. One tablespoon of olive oil should be heated in a big saucepan set over medium heat.

2. Sauté the chopped onion and minced garlic in the saucepan until the onion is tender and transparent. Add the chopped onion to the pot.

3. Add the chopped carrots and celery to the saucepan, then heat for another three to four minutes or until the vegetables have become somewhat softer.

4. Put the lentils that have been rinsed into the pot along with the vegetable broth, diced tomatoes, thyme, smoked paprika, salt, and black pepper. Stir everything together.

5. Bring the mixture to a boil, then immediately decrease the heat to a low setting and allow the soup to simmer for thirty to forty minutes, or until the lentils are soft and the soup has thickened.

6. After the kale leaves have been chopped, add them to the pot and mix everything together.

7. Continue to simmer the soup for five to ten minutes more or until the kale has wilted and become tender.

8. Salt and black pepper should be added to taste after adjusting the seasoning.

9. If you like, you can garnish the Vegetable and Lentil Soup with chopped fresh parsley, a drizzle of olive

oil, or a squeeze of lemon juice and serve it steaming hot.

The preparation of this recipe takes about an hour, and it makes enough food for four servings. While kale is a nutrient-dense leafy green that is rich in vitamins, minerals, and antioxidants, lentils are a good source of plant-based protein and fibre. Lentils also provide a good source of protein. Tomatoes are an excellent food choice for anyone looking to reduce their risk of developing cancer because they contain lycopene and vitamin C.

White Bean and Chicken Chili with Sweet Potato

Ingredients:

One tablespoon of olive oil

One finely sliced onion

three cloves of garlic, minced

1 kilogram of ground chicken; 1 teaspoon of cumin powder

One teaspoon of ground chilli peppers

One teaspoon of oregano that has been dried

One teaspoon of smoked paprika

Two sweet potatoes, peeled and diced

One can of chopped tomatoes, which has not been drained.

One can of white beans, which have been drained and washed.

4 cups of chicken broth with a reduced sodium content

To taste, salt and black pepper will be used.

Additional toppings, if desired: fresh cilantro, shredded cheddar cheese, or sour cream may be added to the dish.

Instructions:

- In a big saucepan that is set over medium heat, warm up one tablespoon of olive oil.
- Sauté the chopped onion and minced garlic in the saucepan until the onion is tender and transparent. Add the chopped onion to the pot.
- Put the ground chicken in the saucepan and cook it over medium heat, breaking it up with a wooden spoon as it cooks until it is browned and fully cooked through.
- To the pot, add the ground cumin, chilli powder, dried oregano, and smoked paprika, and mix to blend all of the spices.
- To the saucepan, add the chopped sweet potatoes, white beans, diced tomatoes, and chicken stock, and mix to blend everything.

- Bring the mixture to a boil, then immediately drop the heat to low and allow the chilli to simmer for thirty to forty minutes, or until the sweet potatoes are soft and the chilli has thickened.

- Salt and black pepper should be added according to taste as you adjust the seasoning.

- If you choose, you can top the White Bean and Chicken Chili with some freshly chopped cilantro, some shredded cheddar cheese, or a dollop of sour cream, and then serve it hot.

- This dish has a total time commitment of around an hour and a half, and it serves six people. Beta-carotene is a potent antioxidant that has been shown to possibly help protect against cancer. Sweet potatoes are a good source of beta-carotene. White beans are an excellent source of fibre as well as protein, and chicken is an excellent choice for a lean supply of protein. This chilli is a tasty and fulfilling way to add cancer-fighting nutrients to your diet, and it's also a great way to get your fill.

A vegetarian dish that is hearty, nutritious, and flavorful, vegetable and quinoa stew is the ideal choice for dining during the fall and winter months. Because it is loaded with cancer-fighting vegetables, protein-rich quinoa, and fragrant spices, it is an excellent choice for individuals who want to increase the amount of cancer-fighting foods they consume in their diet.

quinoa stew made with vegetable

Ingredients:

1 cup quinoa

Two tablespoons of olive oil

One onion, cut into small pieces two cloves of garlic, minced two carrots, cut into small pieces two stalks of celery, cut into small pieces one red bell pepper, cut into small pieces

One can dice tomatoes

4 cups of vegetable broth with a reduced amount of sodium

Two teaspoons of cumin that has been ground

One teaspoon of coriander that has been ground

1/2 teaspoon smoked paprika

Various amounts of salt & pepper, to taste

Parsley, fresh and for the garnish

Directions:

- The quinoa should be washed in cold water and then drained.

- Prepare the sauce by heating the olive oil in a large saucepan over medium heat. Sauté the garlic and onion for a few minutes until they have become more tender.

- After adding the carrots, celery, and red bell pepper, continue to cook the vegetables until they are tender.

- To the pan, add the diced tomatoes, the vegetable broth, the quinoa, the cumin, the coriander, the smoked paprika, and the salt and pepper.

- Bring the mixture to a boil, then reduce the heat and let it simmer for approximately twenty minutes or until the quinoa is completely cooked through.

- Make any necessary adjustments to the seasoning, and sprinkle some fresh parsley on top before serving.

This stew is not only delicious, but it is also an excellent source of fibre, protein, and a variety of different vitamins and minerals. You can eat it as the main course, or you can serve it as a side dish alongside a piece of crusty whole-grain bread.

Chapter 4

Main Dishes

Grilled Salmon with Mango Salsa

Salmon that has been grilled is an excellent main dish that is both tasty and beneficial to one's health because it is loaded with omega-3 fatty acids, protein, and other nutrients that are good for one's body as a whole. This dish would benefit tremendously from the addition of some flavour as well as nutrition if it were served with a mango salsa that was both sweet and sour. The following are the steps to take in order to make grilled salmon with mango salsa:

Ingredients:

Four salmon fillets (6 oz each) (6 oz each)

2 tbsp olive oil

Various amounts of salt and pepper, to taste

One ripe mango, peeled and chopped into small pieces

1/2 of red onion, diced, along with one red bell pepper, diced, and one jalapeno pepper, seeded and chopped.

One lime, squeezed 1/4 cup chopped fresh cilantro

Instructions:

1. Prepare the grill by heating it to a medium-high temperature.
2. Olive oil should be used to coat the salmon fillets before they are seasoned with salt and pepper.
3. Cook the salmon for about four to five minutes with the skin side facing down on the grill.
4. After cooking for an additional two to three minutes on the other side, the salmon should be cooked all the way through.
5. While the salmon is in the oven, make the mango salsa by mixing together a bowl of chopped mango, red onion, red bell pepper, jalapeno pepper, lime juice, and cilantro.
6. Place the grilled salmon on the plate and cover it with the mango salsa.

This meal is not only mouthwatering but it is also loaded with nutrients that may play a role in the prevention and treatment of cancer. Omega-3 fatty acids have been demonstrated to have anti-inflammatory characteristics and may help to lower the risk of some forms of cancer. Salmon is an excellent source of omega-3 fatty acids, which may be found in high concentrations in salmon. In addition, mangoes have a high concentration of antioxidants as well as vitamins A and C, all of which contribute to the maintenance of a healthy immune system.

Chicken with Lemon and Herbs, Roasted, Served with Various Vegetables

A traditional recipe that is both delicious and good for you, lemon and herb roasted chicken with veggies, is a great example. The preparation of a whole supper may be made in a manner that is both simple and delectable by roasting the chicken and veggies simultaneously. The following are the steps to making roasted chicken with lemon, herbs, and vegetables:

Ingredients:

Four drumsticks from a chicken

Four chicken drumsticks

Two tablespoons of olive oil

Various amounts of salt & pepper, to taste

One lemon, peeled and sliced four garlic cloves, peeled and minced one tablespoon of fresh rosemary, chopped one tablespoon of fresh thyme, chopped 1 pound of baby potatoes, cut in half 2 cups of baby carrots

One medium-sized onion, peeled and cut into wedges

Instructions:

- Turn the oven up to 400 degrees Fahrenheit.
- Olive oil, salt, pepper, lemon slices, chopped garlic, rosemary, and thyme should be combined in a bowl and then mixed together.
- In a large baking dish, place chicken thighs and drumsticks.
- After pouring the olive oil mixture over the chicken, make sure it is evenly distributed.
- Place the potatoes, carrots, and onion in the baking dish, then pour any leftover olive oil mixture over the vegetables and toss to coat.

- Bake for 45 to 50 minutes or until the chicken is fully cooked through and the veggies have reached the desired degree of tenderness.

This meal is loaded with ingredients that fight cancer in the body. Chicken is an excellent source of protein and may contribute to the maintenance of an immune system that is healthy. Vitamin C and potassium are just two of the many vitamins and minerals that may be found in abundance in vegetables like carrots and potatoes. In addition, garlic, rosemary, and thyme are all well-known for the antioxidant capabilities that they possess, which aid in preventing cells from being damaged. As part of a well-rounded diet, you should definitely give this delicious and nutritious dinner a try.

Lentil and Sweet Potato Curry

A meal that provides both solace and nourishment, lentil and sweet potato curry is an excellent choice for dining throughout the fall and winter months. Those in search of vegetarian or vegan cooking inspiration may also benefit greatly from this choice. The following is the recipe for the lentil and sweet potato curry:

Ingredients:

1 tbsp coconut oil

One onion, diced

Two cloves of garlic, finely chopped

1 tbsp grated ginger

Two tablespoonfuls of curry powder

1 milligram of ground cumin

1 milligram of coriander seed powder

12 milligrams of ground turmeric

1/4 tsp cayenne pepper (optional)

One sweet potato, peeled and chopped into small pieces

One can (14 oz) diced tomatoes

One can (14 oz) coconut milk

1 cup lentils, either green or brown, that have been dried, rinsed and drained

2 cups of water or broth made from vegetables

Various amounts of salt & pepper, to taste

Fresh cilantro that has been chopped and used as a garnish

Instructions:

1. Warm the coconut oil in a large saucepan or Dutch oven by heating it over medium to high heat.

2. After adding the onion, continue to cook it for about 5 minutes or until it has become soft and translucent.

3. Cook for an additional minute after adding the garlic, ginger, curry powder, cumin, coriander, and turmeric, as well as the cayenne pepper (if using). Cook until the spices release their aroma.

4. Put in the chopped tomatoes, sweet potato, coconut milk, lentils, and water or vegetable broth. Bring the liquid to a boil.

5. Turn the heat down to low, cover the pot, and let it simmer for 25 to 30 minutes, or until the lentils and sweet potatoes are cooked through.

6. Salt and pepper may be added to taste as a seasoning. To serve, bring to a boil and top with chopped fresh cilantro.

This curry made with lentils and sweet potatoes is an excellent source of protein and fibre derived from plants, as well as complex carbs. In addition, lentils are an abundant source of essential vitamins and minerals, including folate, iron, and many others. Beta-carotene is an antioxidant that has been shown to help lower the risk of some forms of cancer. Sweet potatoes have a high concentration of this antioxidant. The fact that this curry is both flavorful and filling makes it an excellent addition to the menu of any person's choice. You can round out your meal with some rice or quinoa if you like.

Chimichurri Sauce Served Over Roasted Cauliflower Steaks.

A delicious and nutritious option for vegetarian main courses is roasted cauliflower steaks drizzled with chimichurri sauce. In addition, they contain few calories and are a rich source of fibre as well as vitamins. This is how you put them together:

Ingredients:

One floret of cauliflower in its head

Two tablespoons of olive oil

Various amounts of salt & pepper, to taste

1/2 cup of fresh parsley that has been chopped

1/4 cup of fresh cilantro that has been chopped

three cloves of garlic, minced

One teaspoon of vinegar made from red wine

1/4 cup olive oil

Various amounts of salt & pepper, to taste

Instructions:

1. Prepare a baking sheet by lining it with parchment paper and preheating the oven to 400 degrees Fahrenheit (200 degrees Celsius).

2. While preserving the cauliflower's stem, cut the vegetable into slices that are 1 inch thick.

3. Olive oil should be used to coat both sides of the cauliflower steaks, and then salt and pepper should be used for seasoning.

4. Roast the cauliflower steaks for 20 to 25 minutes, or until the cauliflower is soft and the steaks have a golden brown colour.

5. As the cauliflower is roasting, you should get started on preparing the chimichurri sauce. Combine the parsley, cilantro, garlic, and garlic powder in a bowl. Add the olive oil, red wine vinegar, and salt and pepper to taste.

6. After it reaches the desired doneness, the cauliflower should be served piping hot with a liberal helping of chimichurri sauce on top.

This recipe is an excellent choice for anyone looking to include more fibre, vitamins, and minerals into their diet. The chimichurri sauce contains herbs that give antioxidants and anti-inflammatory substances, while cauliflower is rich in the vitamins C and K. Folate is also present in significant amounts in cauliflower. Since it is minimal in calories and carbs, this meal is an excellent choice for those who are following a ketogenic or low-carbohydrate diet. The acidic and herbaceous chimichurri sauce adds a punch of flavour to the roasted cauliflower steaks, which already have a pleasant texture thanks to the roasting process. You may either eat it as a main meal or serve it as a side dish with grilled meats or seafood. Both options are delicious.

Chapter 5

Sides and Snacks

Oven-Roasted Broccoli with Garlic and Parmesan

An easy-to-make side dish that is both nutritious and delectable, oven-roasted broccoli with garlic and parmesan cheese is a great option. This dish calls for a limited number of ingredients and can be prepared in less than thirty minutes.

Ingredients:

One broccoli crown, broken Oven-roasted broccoli with garlic and parmesan is a healthy and flavorful side dish that's easy to prepare. This recipe only requires a few ingredients and can be made in under 30 minutes.

Ingredients:

One head of broccoli, cut into florets

Three garlic cloves minced

1/4 cup grated parmesan cheese

Two tablespoons of olive oil

Salt and black pepper to taste

Instructions:

1. Preheat the oven to 400°F (200°C).
2. In a large bowl, toss the broccoli florets with the minced garlic, olive oil, salt, and black pepper until the broccoli is evenly coated.
3. Place the broccoli on a baking sheet in a single layer.
4. Roast the broccoli in the preheated oven for 15-20 minutes or until the edges are crispy and brown.
5. Sprinkle grated parmesan cheese over the broccoli and return the baking sheet to the oven for another 2-3 minutes or until the cheese is melted and bubbly.
6. Serve the roasted broccoli immediately as a healthy side dish. individual florets

three cloves of garlic, minced

Parmesan cheese, grated, one-fourth cup

Two tablespoons of olive oil

To taste, salt and black pepper will be used.

Instructions:

1. Turn the temperature on the oven to 400 degrees Fahrenheit (200 degrees Celsius).
2. the broccoli florets with the minced garlic, olive oil, salt, and black pepper in a large bowl until the broccoli is well covered in the seasoning mixture.
3. Arrange the broccoli in a single layer on a baking pan and set aside.
4. Broccoli should be roasted in an oven that has been warmed for 15 to 20 minutes or until the edges become golden and crispy.
5. On top of the broccoli, sprinkle some grated Parmesan cheese, and then place the baking sheet back into the oven for an additional two to three minutes or until the cheese is melted and bubbling.
6. As a delicious and nutritious side dish, serve the roasted broccoli right away.

Baked Sweet Potato Fries with Rosemary and Sea Salt

Fries made from baked sweet potatoes, seasoned with rosemary and sea salt, make for a snack or side dish that is not only tasty but also beneficial to one's health. This dish calls for a limited number of ingredients and can be prepared in less than thirty minutes.

Ingredients:

2-3 sweet potatoes, depending on their size, peeled and sliced very thinly.
Two tablespoons of olive oil
One tablespoon of fresh rosemary that has been chopped
One teaspoon of sea salt

Instructions:

- Put the oven on to a temperature of 425 degrees Fahrenheit (220 degrees Celsius).
- Sweet potato strips should be tossed in a large basin with olive oil, chopped rosemary, and kosher salt until the sweet potato strips are equally coated with the ingredients.
- On a baking sheet, arrange the sweet potato strips in a single layer.

- Bake the sweet potato fries in an oven that has been warmed for 15 to 20 minutes or until they reach the desired level of crispiness and colour.
- As a tasty and nutritious appetizer or side dish, you may serve the cooked sweet potato fries right away.

Sticks of Cucumber and Carrot with a Yogurt Dipping Sauce

Sticks of cucumber and carrot dipped in yoghurt make for a nutritious and reviving snack that is suitable for consumption at any time of the day. The preparation of this dish is brisk and uncomplicated, and it yields a dish that is abundant in nutritional value.

Ingredients:

One cucumber, peeled and cut into sticks before being sliced.
Around two to three carrots, peeled and cut into sticks.
1 cup of Greek yoghurt in its plain form
One tablespoon of fresh dill that has been chopped
One garlic clove, finely minced

To taste, salt and pepper are available.

Instructions:

- Greek yoghurt, chopped dill, minced garlic, and a pinch each of salt and pepper should be well mixed together in a small basin before proceeding.
- As you are preparing the cucumber and carrot sticks, put the yoghurt dip into the refrigerator to allow it to cool down.
- Sticks of carrots and cucumber should be cut into matchsticks and then arranged on a dish.
- Sticks of cucumber and carrot, together with a cold yoghurt dip, should be served as an appetizer.
- This snack is not only tasty and good for you, but it's also an excellent method for consuming the recommended amount of veggies every day. Enjoy!

Popcorn with Nutritional Yeast and Chili Powder

A tasty and nutritious snack, popcorn that has been seasoned with nutritional yeast and chilli powder is an excellent choice for movie nights or any time you have a need for a savoury snack. This dish is simple to create and may be altered to suit your own tastes in terms of flavour.

Ingredients:

1/2 cup of popcorn hulls and kernels

Two tablespoons of coconut oil

a quarter of a cup of nutritional yeast

1/2 milligram of ground chilli pepper

Salt to taste

Instructions:

- Turn the temperature on in your oven to 375 degrees Fahrenheit.
- Melt the coconut oil in a big saucepan by heating it over medium-high heat until it is completely liquid. Put the lid on the pot once you've added the popcorn kernels to it.
- To prevent the popcorn from becoming burned, shake the pot at regular intervals. Remove the pot from the heat after the popping has slowed to a slower rate, and then let it rest for a minute or two until the popping has entirely ceased.

- Arrange the popcorn in a single layer on a baking sheet that has been covered with parchment paper.
- To make the topping, combine the nutritional yeast, chilli powder, and salt in a small dish.
- The nutritional yeast mixture should be sprinkled over the popcorn and then tossed to get a uniform coating.
- Cook the popcorn in the oven for five to seven minutes, or until the mixture containing the nutritional yeast has become a golden brown colour and the popcorn has become crisp.
- Serve, and have fun with it!

This popcorn is an excellent replacement for the more conventional buttered popcorn, and it is loaded with protein, fibre, and several vitamins. Also, it does not contain any gluten and may be enjoyed by vegans as well as those who are allergic to gluten.

Guacamole with Whole-Grain Chips

Recipe for Guacamole with Chips Made with Whole Grains:

Ingredients:

Two ripe avocados, peeled and pitted, with the pits removed.

a half red onion, cut very finely, one medium tomato, diced

one lime, juiced one-fourth of a cup of fresh cilantro, chopped

To taste, salt and pepper are available.

Tortilla chips made with whole grains

Instructions:

- You may use a potato masher or a fork to mash the avocados in a medium bowl until they are completely smooth.
- To the bowl, add the chopped red onion, diced tomato, lime juice, and chopped cilantro, and toss to blend all of the ingredients.
- Salt and pepper should be added to taste before eating the guacamole.
- To accompany the guacamole, serve tortilla chips made from whole grains.

Note that this guacamole recipe is an excellent choice for a nutritious snack because it is loaded with flavour and healthy fats. While avocado provides monounsaturated fats that are good for the heart, whole-grain chips are a good source of fibre.

Chapter 6

Desserts and Treats

Berry and Yogurt Popsicles

Popsicles made with yoghurt and berries make for a sweet treat that is both tasty and good for you—just what you need when the temperature starts to rise. They are simple to prepare and may be altered to suit your own tastes in terms of flavour. You may use fresh or frozen berries, yoghurt, and whatever kind of sweetener you choose in these homemade popsicles.

Ingredients:

2 cups of assorted berries, either fresh or frozen (such as strawberries, raspberries, and blueberries)
One standard serving size of plain Greek yoghurt

Two tablespoons of honey, or maple syrup, whatever you choose (or to taste)

Popsicle moulds

Instructions:

- Blend or process the berries in a food processor or blender until they reach a creamy consistency.
- In a separate dish, thoroughly blend the yoghurt and sweetener so that they form a single substance.
- Add the yoghurt mixture and the berry puree to the popsicle moulds in alternating layers until they are completely filled.
- After inserting the popsicle sticks, place the moulds in the freezer for at least four hours or until the contents are totally frozen.
- To free the popsicles from their moulds, just submerge them in warm water for a few seconds before attempting to remove them.

These Berry and Yogurt Popsicles are an excellent choice for a nutritious dessert since they include both antioxidants and protein in abundant amounts.

Chocolate Avocado Pudding

Ingredients

Two ripe avocados, peeled and pitted, with the pits removed.

a quarter of a cup of cocoa powder, unsweetened

1/4 cup maple syrup

1 tsp vanilla extract 1/4 cup almond milk

Instructions:

- Put the avocado, cocoa powder, maple syrup, and vanilla extract in a food processor or a blender and process until smooth.
- After adding the almond milk, continue blending until the mixture is silky smooth.
- As a dessert that is both wholesome and satisfying, serve it chilled.

Baked Apples with Cinnamon and Walnuts

Ingredients:

Two apples, cored and sliced with their skins on

1 milligram of cinnamon

1/4 cup of walnuts that have been chopped

1 tbsp maple syrup

1 tsp vanilla extract

Instructions:

- Preheat the oven to 375 degrees Fahrenheit.
- Spread the apple slices out in the bottom of a baking dish.
- Cinnamon, chopped walnuts, maple syrup, and vanilla essence should all be combined in a small basin and stirred together.
- The cinnamon mixture should be sprinkled on top of the cut apples.
- Bake the apples for 20 to 25 minutes or until they reach the desired consistency.
- Serve warm as a nutritious and delicious alternative to traditional desserts.

Take note: these recipes for sweets and snacks are nutritious alternatives that will sate your want for something sweet while also supplying your body with essential nutrients. These are wonderful for those who want to treat themselves to something sweet but don't want to jeopardize their efforts to improve their health.

Chocolate and Peanut Butter Energy Balls

Recipe for Energy Balls made with Chocolate and Peanut Butter:

Ingredients:

1 cup of traditional rolled oats (old-fashioned)
1/2 cup creamy peanut butter
a quarter of a cup of honey, a quarter of a cup of unsweetened cocoa powder
1/4 cup of tiny chocolate chips
1/4 cup of peanuts that have been chopped
1/4 tsp salt

Directions:

- Mix the peanut butter, honey, cocoa powder, micro chocolate chips, chopped peanuts, and salt together in a large bowl. Add the rolled oats and mix well. Mix until everything is evenly distributed.

- The mixture has to be allowed to cool and become hard for approximately half an hour before it can be used, so cover the bowl and put it in the refrigerator.
- When the dough has been cold, scoop it out using a cookie scoop or a spoon and then shape it into balls. Arrange the balls in a single layer on a baking sheet that has been covered with parchment paper.
- To let the balls harden into their final form, return the baking sheet to the refrigerator with its cover on for an additional half an hour.
- After they have hardened, you can keep the energy balls in the refrigerator for up to a week in an airtight container.

These energy balls are an excellent snack for sustained energy as well as a sweet treat without the added sugar since they are filled with protein, fibre, and healthy fats.

Coconut Milk Pudding with Fresh Fruit

Individuals who are seeking a sweet treat that does not include any added sugar will appreciate the nutritious and delectable qualities of the Coconut Milk Pudding with Fresh Fruit. Since it calls for coconut milk rather than dairy milk, this dish is an excellent choice for anyone who is lactose intolerant or who follows a diet that does not include dairy products.

Ingredients:

One tin of coconut milk with all the fat

1/4 cup chia seeds

One tablespoon of maple syrup or honey

1 tsp vanilla extract

Fresh fruit is to be used as a topping.

Instructions:

- Coconut milk, chia seeds, honey or maple syrup, and vanilla essence should be mixed together in a bowl using a whisk until the ingredients are well incorporated.
- After allowing the mixture to rest for ten to fifteen minutes, whisk it once more to break up any clumps that may have formed.
- Place the mixture in individual serving cups and chill it in the refrigerator for at least two hours or for as long as overnight.

- Before serving, top each portion with a piece of the fresh fruit of your choosing.

You may adjust the amount of honey or maple syrup you use, depending on how sweet you want it, and you can try out a variety of fruits to use as toppings. This recipe is quite versatile and easy to adapt to your own tastes in terms of flavour. This satiating and wholesome dessert is made possible by the use of coconut milk and chia seeds, both of which are good sources of fibre and healthy fats.

Chapter 7

Fruits and Vegetables

Fruits and vegetables are not only necessary components of a diet that is healthy, but they also have the potential to be very effective in the fight against cancer. They are chock-full of antioxidants, vitamins, and minerals, all of which assist in promoting immune function and fighting free radicals, the presence of which has been linked to an increased risk of developing cancer. Consuming a wide range of fruits and vegetables may assist in the maintenance of a healthy weight, which is another element that plays a significant role in the prevention of cancer.

The following are some of the most beneficial fruits and vegetables for preventing cancer:

- Berries, including blueberries, strawberries, raspberries, and blackberries, are jam-packed with antioxidants and other substances that research has shown to have anti-cancer qualities.

- Cruciferous veggies: Broccoli, cauliflower, Brussels sprouts, and kale are all members of the same family of plants known as cruciferous vegetables. These vegetables include substances that have been associated with a decreased risk of developing cancer.

- Leafy greens: Spinach, kale, Swiss chard, and other leafy greens are abundant in cancer-fighting minerals such as folate, vitamin C, and beta-carotene. These nutrients have all been demonstrated to have anti-cancer qualities.

- Tomatoes: Tomatoes are an excellent source of the potent antioxidant known as lycopene, which has been associated with a lower risk of numerous different forms of cancer.

- Oranges, grapefruits, lemons, and limes are all rich sources of vitamin C, which has been associated with a lower risk of cancer. Other citrus fruits, such as lemons and limes, are also strong sources of vitamin C.

It is possible to include a wide range of fruits and vegetables into your diet in a way that is not only simple but also tasty. You may want to experiment by including berries in your morning smoothie, munching on carrot sticks and hummus in the afternoon, or cooking a pan full of mixed veggies for supper. There is no justifiable excuse for excluding fruits and vegetables from one's diet, given the wide variety of scrumptious and wholesome preparations from which one might select.

The combination of beets and carrots produces a juice that is both reviving and wholesome since it is rich in vitamins and antioxidants. You need fresh beets and carrots, in addition to a juicer, in order to prepare this juice.

Ingredients:

Two medium-sized beets have been cleaned and trimmed.

Four medium-sized carrots have been cleaned and trimmed.

Instructions:

- Be sure to cut the beets and carrots into bite-sized pieces before placing them in the juicer.
- Be sure to follow the directions provided by the manufacturer while juicing the beets and carrots.
- Mix the juice, and serve it as soon as possible.

Consuming a glass of juice made from beets and carrots is an excellent approach to getting the vitamins and antioxidants you need on a daily basis. Although carrots are abundant in vitamin A, vitamin K, and potassium, beets are an excellent source of folate and manganese. Potassium, vitamin A, and vitamin K are also present in beets. This juice is also an excellent source of dietary fibre, which may play an important role in maintaining a healthy digestive tract. Include a serving of this scrumptious and healthful juice in your regular routine of eating.

This green vegetable may be enjoyed in a manner that is both tasty and beneficial to one's diet by grilling it with lemon and garlic. The vegetable known as asparagus is loaded with a variety of essential vitamins and minerals, such as vitamins A,

C, E, and K, in addition to folate and potassium. This extremely healthful vegetable receives an additional boost in taste and antioxidant capacity when grilled with lemon and garlic.

To begin preparing this meal, clip the woody ends off of your asparagus stalks and set them aside. They should be seasoned with salt and pepper and drizzled with olive oil before serving. After that, place them on the grill and cook them over medium-high heat for three to five minutes on each side or until they are cooked and have a little sear.

While the asparagus is on the grill, you may make the sauce with lemon and garlic. In a small bowl, combine the minced garlic with the juice of one-half of a lemon, one tablespoon of olive oil, and a sprinkle of salt and pepper, and stir to combine. As soon as the asparagus reaches the desired doneness, quickly pour the lemon and garlic sauce over the top, and then serve. This meal is delicious when served as a side to grilled meats or seafood, but it also stands well on its own as a savoury and nutritious snack on its own.

Roasted Sweet Potato and Kale Salad

The Roasted Sweet Potato and Kale Salad is salad that is excellent for any occasion since it is both tasty and healthful. It is topped with a zesty lemon vinaigrette and is loaded with nutritious vegetables such as roasted sweet potato, kale, and quinoa.

Ingredients:

Two sweet potatoes, peeled and cut into cubes of medium size
One bunch of kale, with the stems removed and the leaves ripped into bite-sized pieces
1 ounce of ready-to-eat quinoa
1/4 cup of feta cheese in crumbled form
1/4 cup of walnuts that have been chopped
Cranberries, dry, one-fourth cup
1/4 cup olive oil
Two teaspoons of lemon juice
One garlic clove, finely minced
To taste, salt and pepper are available.

Directions:

- Turn the oven up to 400 degrees Fahrenheit.

- Cut the sweet potatoes into cubes and place them on a baking pan that has been coated with parchment paper. Salt and pepper should also be added once the olive oil has been drizzled on top. Roast in the oven for 20 to 25 minutes or until the vegetables are soft and have a light browning.

- When the sweet potatoes are roasting, get the kale ready by rubbing it with olive oil to soften it up. This may be done while the sweet potatoes are cooking. Put aside.

- To create the dressing, put the olive oil, lemon juice, minced garlic, salt, and pepper into a small bowl and whisk all of the ingredients together.

- Combine the roasted sweet potatoes, kale that has been massaged, quinoa that has been cooked, crumbled feta cheese, chopped walnuts, and dried cranberries in a large bowl.

- After drizzling the lemon vinaigrette over the salad, mix the ingredients together in a low-key manner.

- Serve the salad right away, or put it in the refrigerator until you are ready to serve it.

This salad is an excellent choice for a wholesome and satiating main course or side dish alternative. A range of nutrients is provided by the combination of roasted sweet potatoes, quinoa, and kale, and the addition of zesty lemon vinaigrette offers a taste that is energizing and revitalizing. Enjoy!

Conclusion

Final Thoughts on Cancer-Fighting Recipes and Lifestyle Changes

In conclusion, it is essential to keep in mind that leading a healthy lifestyle may significantly contribute to the reduction of the risk of developing cancer. If you want to improve your general health and sense of well-being, it may be beneficial to make a few simple adjustments to your diet on a regular basis, such as eating more fruits and vegetables. You may take the first step toward a better lifestyle and minimize your chance of acquiring cancer by making use of the recipes in this guide that fight cancer. These recipes are offered for your convenience.

In addition to maintaining a healthy diet, practising stress reduction methods and engaging in regular physical exercise are all important components of an effective cancer prevention practice. You may take charge of your health and lower your chance of developing cancer by implementing the aforementioned adjustments to your lifestyle.

It is essential to remember that adopting a healthy diet and way of life may reduce the chance of developing cancer, but it does not ensure that the disease will be completely avoided. Cancer screenings on a regular basis and early diagnosis are both very important steps in the process of locating and treating cancer in its earlier stages.

You may take charge of your health and well-being by adopting a proactive stance toward it and combining healthy behaviours with routine checkups. Keep in mind that even little adjustments may have a significant impact on the promotion of a healthy lifestyle and the reduction of the risk of developing cancer.

There are many more resources available to assist you in making healthy decisions and lowering your risk of developing cancer, in addition to the recipes and suggestions that are offered in this guide. Listed below are some ideas to consider:

- The American Institute for Cancer Research (AICR) is a charitable organization whose mission is to reduce the risk of cancer via increased awareness, research, and education. The American Institute for Cancer Research (AICR) provides a multitude of materials on healthy eating and active lifestyles, such as meal planning, recipes, and advice for grocery shopping.

- The National Cancer Institute (NCI) is a government institution that carries out cancer research and provides financial assistance for it. The National Cancer Institute (NCI) offers a variety of materials on healthy living, such as recommendations for good eating and physical exercise, recipes, and guidance for cancer survivors.

- The Global Cancer Research Fund International is an organization that has a primary emphasis on the prevention of cancer via dietary choices, proper nutrition, and regular exercise. This website provides advice based on science, as well as recipes and ideas for living a healthy lifestyle.

- Local health groups: A great number of towns and cities have local organizations whose only mission is to encourage healthy living and illness prevention. In order to find out what options are offered in your region, you can contact the health department or cancer centre in your area.

You may lower your risk of cancer and improve your general health by making some simple adjustments to your food and the way you live your life. You may begin your path toward a better and happier life by using the recipes and resources that are offered in this book as a beginning point on your trip.